EXPERT SECRETS FOR A STRESS-FREE, FUN AND AMAZING FIRST TIME MOM AND DAD

THE SIMPLIFIED APPROACH TO YOUR FIRST PREGNANCY JOURNEY.

BY:

JOYNER WILLIAMS

TABEL OF CONTENTS

INTRODUCTION

As stunning as it may be, turning into a parent unexpectedly has its difficulties: You're exploring a significant life change on little rest and without the advantage of involvement. However, you change, your certainty develops and the stretches of rest around evening time broaden—and you may before long feel ready for growing your family once more.

At the point when you do, don't be astounded if everything feels less extraordinary. Science demonstrates turning into a mother unexpectedly is commonly more extraordinary both actually and genuinely than the involvement in later youngsters. First-time parenthood is so difficult on the grounds that it's simply so new. Irrespective of your budget, it is so unlikely you can completely accommodate all that comes along with it.

In this book, I will take you on a very simplified journey as a first mom and dad, and I promise you won't be left stranded following this guide.

CHAPTER ONE

New mothers go through 1,400 hours of internet investigating approaches to keep their infants upbeat and solid. This stressing goes with the job of encountering an entirely different sort of obligation.

Turning out to be pregnant is just the start however it's an imperative stage in your kid's wellbeing. Start in good shape by following these ten hints for first-time pregnancies.

1. Keep away from Caffeine

Drinking caffeine during pregnancy has some significant health risks. The caffeine gets processed much increasingly slow through the placenta into your infant's circulation system. This implies that the caffeine results to a dashing pulse, hypertension, and an invigorated sensory system that can influence you and your child. The outcome is a higher possibility of an unnatural birth cycle. Indeed, even limited quantities have been known to cause a 13% expansion in low birth weight for your infant.

Have a goal at changing to a normally decaffeinated natural tea, yet consult   your PCP or birthing assistant as specific spices can cause untimely labor.

2. Exercise Regularly

Having an infant is both physically and mentally demanding. To battle the agony and emotional episodes that accompany being pregnant, practice routinely. Low effect exercise can help move back torment, increase blood circulation, and improve your disposition. It will likewise reinforce your muscles and tendons in anticipation of work.

Incorporate some incredible activities that limit the weight on you such as swimming and strolling. Yoga expands ripeness rates and pre-birth yoga opens up your hips, mitigates pressure, and helps with eagerness. Lifting weighty loads or debilitating yourself through extraordinary cardio exercises may accomplish more damage than anything else.

3. Drink Plenty of Water

First-time mothers require more water than ordinary as it turns out to be essential for the amniotic liquid that encompasses your infant. The low liquid can prompt premature delivery or birth defects. You can get dehydrated quickly while pregnant since you need more than you are accustomed to. It is suggested that you drink in any event 10 cups of 8 ounces every day to remain hydrated.

Drinking enough water can likewise mitigate swollen joints and flush your organs of developed poisons.

4. Take Naps

Weakness, particularly during the primary trimester, is normal. Your body is experiencing hormonal changes that will influence your energy levels. Take the time presently to get up to speed with rest and let your body unwind. When the child is born, you won't have the occasion to rest as frequently. Your rest timetable will be conflicting and lacking. Thus, treat yourself to an evening snooze to reestablish yourself and help facilitate the pressure of work and individual life on your child. Getting the perfect measure of rest around evening time is additionally significant. As your pregnancy advances, it will turn out to be harder to rest around the evening time. You will utilize the washroom frequently and battle to locate an agreeable situation for your bump. Compensate for lost rest around evening time and get yourself a pregnancy cushion that goes in the middle of your thighs and under your beneath. A cushion will adjust your hips to ease the heat away from you and the pelvis.

5. Pre-birth Massage

Prior to conceiving an offspring, plan a period for an expert pre-birth rub. A low-sway massage treats lower back agony that can be a threat all through your pregnancy. It will likewise expand dissemination and eliminate aggravation that causes growing. Maintain a strategic distance from a back rub toward the start of your first trimester. Most specialists won't acknowledge ladies during this time as the opportunity of premature delivery is higher. You can get a massage whenever up into your due date after that.

6. Make a Birth Arrangement

Being a mother starts during the birth of your infant. You need to make this second exceptional and safe. That is the reason making a birthing arrangement is basic. Do your own examination online about your alternatives prior to taking any guidance from loved ones. This is your choice so you ought to have an impartial perspective on the approach. While a medical clinic birth is conventional, an ascent in the utilization of maternity specialists and even home births are happening in the USA. There has been a 77% expansion in home birth from 2004 to 2017. Your area isn't the main decision you need to make. The choices to utilize an epidural, have a water birth, or a postponed line clasping are only a couple more.

7. Go Out on the town to shop

Get energized for your beloved newborn by getting those fundamental and adorable child things prepared. You can set up the nursery with a bunk, evolving table, rocker, and dresser. Also, select a brilliant tone for the dividers and decals for the windows for your infant to appreciate. Dressing your child is fun, yet it requires a great deal of arranging. You would prefer not to run out of garments when your child has a development spray. Plan to get one size up from their present age. Infant garments won't keep going long so just purchase a couple. You additionally need to settle on diaper marks or pick a fabric or reusable supplements. For infants, expendable diapers work the best since you will be changing all the time. As they get more seasoned, you may change to a more eco-accommodating alternative. Remember about covers, napkins, jugs, and some starter toys. These things will assist you with getting ready both physically and mentally.

8. Travel Smart

Proceed, book that flight, however, avoid potential risk. The Mayo Clinic says mid-pregnancy (14 to 28 weeks) is typically the best opportunity to fly—at this point you're most likely over with morning sickness, and the danger of premature labor is slow. In any case, check with your primary care physician about any itinerary items, and ensure the aircraft has no limitations for pregnant ladies. On the plane, drink a lot of water to remain hydrated, and get up and stroll around each half-hour to decrease the danger of blood clumps. A path seat will give you more space and make outings to the washroom simpler. In the vehicle, keep on wearing a seat strap. As indicated by the National Highway Traffic Safety Administration, the shoulder segment of the restriction ought to be situated over the collar bone. The lap bit ought to be put under the midsection as low as conceivable on the hips and over the upper thighs, never over the mid-region. Additionally, pregnant ladies ought to sit as a long way from the airbag as could reasonably be expected

9. Wear Sunscreen

Being pregnant makes your skin more touchy to daylight, so you're more inclined to burn from the sun and chloasma, those dull smeared spots that occasionally show up on the face. Apply a sunscreen with an SPF of 30 or higher (numerous brands presently offer compound free equations synthetic-free) and wear a cap and shades. While no examinations demonstrate investing energy in tanning beds can hurt your infant, the American Pregnancy Association suggests you stay away from them while you're pregnant.

10. Track Your Weight Gain

We know—you're eating for two. Yet, pressing on such a large number of additional pounds may make them difficult to lose later. Simultaneously, not increasing enough can put the child in danger for a low-weight birth, a significant reason for formative issues. As of late, the Institute of Medicine (IOM) gave new rules for weight gain during pregnancy. This is what the IOM suggests, in light of a lady's BMI (weight file) prior to getting pregnant with one infant:

- Underweight: Gain 28-40 pounds

- Normal weight: Gain 25-35 pounds

- Overweight: Gain 15-25 pounds

- Obese: Gain 11-20 pounds

Book appointment with your primary care physician often to ensure you're picking up at a sound rate

CHAPTER 2

10 Things Soon-To-Be-Dads Should Know About Pregnant Women

You will be a father—congrats! These tips, stunts, and rules will assist you with confronting first-time parenthood.

1. Yearnings

Yearnings are genuine. She will presumably have numerous desires all through her pregnancy. Keep her cheerful by going to get those fries or chocolate at 10 p.m. It may be somewhat badly arranged for you, however, it will fulfill her. An upbeat spouse is a cheerful life.

2. Infant Weight

Ladies will regularly increase 25-35 pounds during their pregnancy. It is significant that you understand that you are not putting on child weight with her. You are not conveying an infant, so there is no explanation behind you to gain extra weight with your pregnant spouse. She is consuming a lot of extra calories, so she needs to eat more. Be that as it may, you are not needing additional calories. It may be hard with all the additional shoddy nourishment lying around, yet it will be significantly harder to lose that gut fat you picked up.

3. Tired

She will most likely become tired in light of the fact that she is developing another life inside her. Her body is working diligently rolling out the essential improvements to oblige your infant. She may likewise encounter anxious rest, making her be more drained. Recall that she is worn out. Do some additional things around the house. Convey the clothing bin up the steps or prepare the dinner while she rests.

4. Continuous Urination

An indication of pregnancy is heading off to the washroom, a ton. Getting up a few times for the duration of the night to utilize the restroom will turn into everyday practice for her. That 2-hour vehicle ride without any stops will transform into a 2 and 15-minute vehicle ride with two stops. She's disturbed about it either, so no whining from your end.

5. Bunches Of Pillows

There will be a ton of cushions that begin showing up on your bed. As expected, you may find that there is no space for you any longer. For this situation, we trust you have an agreeable love seat. Your pregnant spouse may encounter slow posture changes to acclimate to the pregnancy weight. This can bring about strain, causing back torment. Cushions can help reduce this torment. She will most likely be snuggling with a giant body pillow rather than you. Try not to think about it literally, she is simply attempting to get as agreeable as could reasonably be expected.

6. A throbbing painfulness

Since her body is extending, moving, and moving everywhere , there will undoubtedly be a throbbing painfulness. She is conveying the extra weight that her body needs to help. This additional weight will cause weight on the lower back. Back rubs are an extraordinary help for her toward the day's end. Back rubs all in all are an absolute necessity for pregnant ladies. Regardless of whether they are foot, back, or hip back rubs, you must assist her out calm however much strain as could be expected.

7. Heightened Sensory

Your spouse might have very heightened sensory during her pregnancy, including her feeling of smell. It seems like good judgment however, on the other hand you'd help her to abstain from eating things she's delicate to. Even while you're not together, as you will get back home possessing a scent like whatever is more perceptible to her. It might appear to be a troublesome thing to oblige, in any event, staying away from things while you're not together, but rather she'll see your eagerness to make things as simple on her as could be expected under the circumstances and will most likely value it.

8. Stresses

It is very normal for both of you to have stress over how your own life and life as a team will change with a child. Set aside the effort to converse with your spouse about the forthcoming changes, a bit at a time. (12 PM probably won't be the best time, however.) Use this pregnancy time to search out the opinion of your trusted and experienced companions, your primary care physician, even your folks. Think about everybody's recommendation while taking other factors into consideration – each family circumstance is one of a kind.

9. Your relationship

There's no rejecting that thinking about an infant can be debilitating. Following a month or so you may be feeling drained, focused, and overpowered. You may likewise be discovering you have various thoughts from your spouse about how to be a parent. Conversing with one another and tuning in to one another's perspective is the most ideal approach to conquer these sentiments. It is best for your child in the event that you parent as a group, where you settle on choices together, consent to your parts as guardians, and manage struggle tranquility and deferentially.

Sexual connections can change after the birth of a child as well. Moms are likely prompted not to engage in sexual relations until after their 6-week postnatal routine. That being said, a child's mom may discover sex uninteresting due to actual changes after birth, or even postnatal gloom.

On the off chance that your spouse is the mother, showing restraint toward her while she is recuperating, discovering different approaches to be cozy (like kissing and snuggling), and assisting in child care and family tasks will keep your bond solid.

10. Taking care of yourself

With all that is going on, it tends to be anything but difficult to disregard caring for yourself. Eating soundly, doing some actual movement, and attempting to get enough rest is immeasurably essential to keep your energy step up. Keep in mind, fathers, get postnatal uneasiness and sadness as well. On the off chance that you are feeling drained, fractious, or furious, on the off chance that you feel overpowered or that you can't adapt, it's imperative to get counsel from your primary care physician. It can take mental fortitude to look for help – however, it's the best thing you can accomplish for your family.

CHAPTER THREE

A baby moon is basically a casual escape for hopeful moms and their spouse before their fresh newborn moves in! It has become an undeniably developing pattern for mums-to-be to take off on vacation with either their spouse, or a friend or family member before the unavoidable satisfaction of the newborn. A few couples decide to go on a baby moon as their 'last' occasion as only a couple preceding their change into having a family.

It is critical to take note that baby moons are frequently taken in the second trimester of pregnancy after the 12-week check up, then it is a lot more secure in the event that you need to fly out. On the off chance that you need to travel to another country for your baby moon or are thinking about a long stretch flight it is consistently prudent to seek the advice of your clinical specialist.

Flying out before the 12 weeks of pregnancy isn't fitting; be that as it may, on the off chance that you truly need to go on a baby moon before 12 weeks you could consider a neighborhood spa excursion or loosened up inn remain. All get-away plans ought to be considered in accordance with your individual wellbeing and necessities as it's essential to remain fit and solid while being pregnant. You may wish to consider what sort of protection you wish to take and might need to talk about your arrangements with your birthing specialist.

On the off chance that you are thinking about where to go for your baby moon there is a scope of objections to browse. Most couples need to invest some loosening up energy off in relaxed environment before the restless evenings start. From stunning sea shores to loosened up spa ends of the week or a lavish inn remain, there are a wide range of spots that you could decide to make the most of your baby moon.

On the off chance that you are on edge or stressed over going anyplace abroad you might need to attempt alternatives, for example, having a pre-birth knead, setting off to the theater, appreciating some top notch food, or have a lavish inn end of the week remain.

On the off chance that you like nature and appreciate respecting the greenery why not book into a field resort or absorb some daylight at the sea shore. There are numerous objections that have ocean side inns that you can appreciate and on the off chance that you are feeling peckish you could utilize the fish.

Another alternative for the individuals who want to go on a short-pull flight is to pick a city break. You can appreciate the way of life and history of the absolute most dynamic urban communities in Europe and some movement administrators permit you to visit two urban areas while booking to go to one.

On the off chance that you are truly audacious and have the support from your birthing assistant to fly out long stretch you might need to think about a fascinating sea shore area, or a daylight resort.

CHAPTER FOUR

Inside 24 hours after fertilization, the egg that will end up being your infant quickly partitions into numerous cells. By the eighth day stretch of pregnancy, your child will change names from an embryo to fetus. There are around 40 weeks to a run of the mill pregnancy. These weeks are isolated into three trimesters. Find out about your child's advancement all through each phase of pregnancy.

When does a pregnancy start

The beginning of pregnancy is really the primary day of your last feminine period. This is known as the gestational age, or feminine age. It's around fourteen days in front of when conception really happens. Despite the fact that it might appear to be bizarre, the date of the principal day of your last period will be a significant date while deciding your infant's expected date. Your medical services supplier will get some information about this date and will utilize it to sort out how far along you are in your pregnancy.

Every month, your body experiences a regenerative cycle that can end in one of two different ways. You will either have a feminine period or gotten pregnant. This cycle is constantly occurring during your conceptive years—from pubescence in your adolescent years to menopause around age 50.

In a cycle that closes with pregnancy, there are a few stages. Initial, a gathering of eggs (called oocytes) prepares to leave the ovary for ovulation (arrival of the egg). The eggs create in little, liquid filled pimples called follicles. Consider these follicles as little holders for each youthful egg. Out of this gathering of eggs, one will get developed and proceed through the cycle. This follicle at that point smothers the wide range of various follicles in the gathering. Different follicles quit developing now.

The develop follicle presently opens and delivers the egg from the ovary. This is ovulation. Ovulation for the most part occurs around fourteen days before your next feminine period starts. It's for the most part in the center of your cycle.

After ovulation, the opened (cracked) follicle forms into a structure called the corpus luteum. This secretes (discharges) the hormones progesterone and estrogen. The progesterone readies the endometrium (covering of the uterus). This coating, is where a treated egg settles to create. In the event that you don't get pregnant during a cycle, this covering is what is shed during your period.

By and large, treatment occurs around fourteen days after your last feminine period. At the point when the sperm enters the egg, changes happen in the protein covering of the egg to keep other sperm from entering.

Right now of treatment, your infant's hereditary make-up is finished, including its sex. The sexual orientation of your child relies upon what sperm treats the egg right now of origination. By and large, ladies have a hereditary blend of XX and men have XY. As the mother, you furnish each egg with a X. Every sperm can be either a X or a Y. In the event that the treated egg and sperm is a mix of a X and Y, it's a kid. In the event that there are two Xs, it's a young lady.

What happens just after conception?
Inside 24 hours after preparation, the egg starts quickly partitioning into numerous cells. It stays in the fallopian tube for around three days after origination. At that point, the treated egg (presently called a blastocyte) keeps on separating as it goes gradually through the fallopian cylinder to the

uterus. Once there, its next employment is to join to the endometrium. This is called implantation.

Prior to implantation, however, the blastocyte breaks out of its defensive covering. At the point when the blastocyte connects with the endometrium, the two trade hormones to enable the blastocyte to append. A few ladies notice spotting (slight seeping) during a couple of days when implantation occurs. This is typical and isn't something you should stress over. Now, the endometrium gets thicker and the cervix (the opening between your uterus and birth channel) is fixed by an attachment of bodily fluid.

Inside three weeks, the blastocyte cells at last structure a little ball, or an undeveloped organism. At this point, the infant's first nerve cells have shaped.

Your creating child has just experienced a couple of name changes in the initial barely any long stretches of pregnancy. By and large, your child will be called an undeveloped organism from origination until the eighth seven day stretch of improvement. After the eighth week, the child will be known as a fetus until it's conceived.

From the snapshot of origination, the hormone human chorionic gonadotrophin (hCG) will be available in your blood. This hormone is made by the cells that structure the placenta (food hotspot for your infant in the belly). It's likewise the hormone distinguished in a pregnancy test. Despite the fact that this hormone is there from the earliest starting point, it takes effort for it to work inside your body. It regularly takes three to about a month from the principal day of your last period for the hCG to build enough to be recognized by pregnancy tests.

When would it be a good idea for me to connect with my medical services supplier about another pregnancy?

Most medical care suppliers will have you stand by to come in for an arrangement until you have had a positive home pregnancy test. These tests are precise once you have enough hCG flowing all through your body. This can be half a month after origination. It's ideal to call your medical services supplier once you have a positive pregnancy test to plan your first arrangement.

At the point when you call, your medical care supplier may inquire as to whether you are taking a pre-birth nutrient. These enhancements contain something many refer to as folic corrosive. It's significant that you get at any rate 400mcg of folic corrosive every day during pregnancy to ensure your child's neural cylinder (start of the infant's mind and spine) grows accurately. Numerous medical services suppliers recommend that you take pre-birth nutrients with folic corrosive in any event, when you aren't pregnant. On the off chance that you weren't taking pre-birth nutrients before your pregnancy, your supplier may request that you start as right on time as could reasonably be expected.

What's The Course Of Events For My Infant's Turn Of Events?

Your infant will change a ton all through an ordinary pregnancy. This time is separated into three phases, called trimesters. Every trimester is a bunch of around a quarter of a year. Your medical services supplier will most likely converse with you about your infant's advancement regarding weeks. In this way, in the event that you are three months pregnant, you are around 12 weeks. You will see unmistakable changes in your infant, and yourself, during every trimester.

Generally, we consider a pregnancy a nine-month measure. In any case, this isn't generally the situation. A full-term pregnancy is 40 weeks or 280 days. Contingent upon what months you are pregnant during (some are more limited and some more) and what week you convey, you could be pregnant for either nine months or 10 months. This is totally ordinary and solid.

When you draw near to the furthest limit of your pregnancy, there are a few classification names you may hear with respect to when you start giving birth. These marks split the most recent couple of long stretches of pregnancy. They're likewise used to pay special mind to specific difficulties in infants. Infants that are conceived in the early term time frame or before may have a higher danger of breathing, hearing, or learning issues than children brought into the world half a month later in the full-term time period. At the point when you're taking a gander at these marks, it's critical to realize how they're composed. You may see the week initial (38) and afterward, you'll see two numbers isolated by a slice mark (6/7). This represents how long you as of now are in the gestational week. Along these lines, in the event that you see 38 6/7, it implies that you are on day 6 of your 38th week.

The most recent couple of long stretches of pregnancy are separated into the accompanying gatherings:

- **Early term**: 37 0/7 weeks through 38 6/7 weeks.
- **Full term**: 39 0/7 weeks through 40 6/7 weeks.
- **Late term**: 41 0/7 weeks through 41 6/7 weeks.

Post term: 42 0/7 weeks and on

Converse with your medical services supplier about any inquiries you may have about your child's gestational age and due date.

CHAPTER FIVE

First trimester

The main trimester will length from origination to 12 weeks. This is commonly the initial three months of pregnancy. During this trimester, your infant will transform from a little gathering of cells to a hatchling that is beginning to have a child's highlights.

Month 1 (weeks 1 through 4)

As the treated egg grows, a water-tight sac structures around it, step by step loading up with liquid. This is known as the amniotic sac, and it helps pad the developing undeveloped organism.

During this time, the placenta additionally creates. The placenta is a round, level organ that moves supplements from the mother to the infant, and moves squanders from the child. Consider the placenta a food hotspot for your child all through the pregnancy.

In these initial hardly any weeks, a crude face will take structure with huge dark circles for eyes. The mouth, lower jaw and throat are creating. Platelets are coming to fruition, and course will start. The minuscule "heart" cylinder will thump 65 times each moment before the finish of the fourth week.

Before the finish of the primary month, your infant is around 1/4 inch long – more modest than a grain of rice.

Month (fourteen days 5 through 8)

Your child's facial highlights keep on creating. Every ear starts as a little overlay of skin along the edge of the head. Small buds that inevitably develop into arms and legs are shaping. Fingers, toes and eyes are additionally framing.

The neural cylinder (mind, spinal rope and other neural tissue of the focal sensory system) is all around framed at this point. The stomach related parcel and tangible organs start to grow as well. Bone begins to supplant ligament. Your child's head is enormous in relation to the remainder of its body now. At around a month and a half, your infant's heart beat can generally be distinguished.

After the eighth week, your child is known as a hatchling rather than an undeveloped organism. Before the second's over month, your child is around 1 inch long and weighs around 1/30 of an ounce.

Month 3 (weeks 9 through 12)

Your child's arms, hands, fingers, feet and toes are full grown. At this stage, your infant is beginning to investigate a piece by doing things like opening and shutting its clench hands and mouth. Fingernails and toenails are starting to create and the outer ears are shaped. The beginnings of teeth are shaping under the gums. Your child's regenerative organs additionally grow, however the infant's sexual orientation is hard to recognize on ultrasound.

Before the finish of the third month, your infant is full fledged. All the organs and appendages (furthest points) are available and will keep on creating so as to get utilitarian. The child's circulatory and urinary frameworks are additionally working and the liver produces bile. Toward the finish of the third month, your infant is around 4 inches in length and weighs around 1 ounce.

Since your infant's most basic advancement has occurred, your possibility of unnatural birth cycle drops significantly following three months.

Second trimester

This center segment of pregnancy is regularly considered as the best piece of the experience. At this point, any morning affliction is most likely gone and the uneasiness of early pregnancy has blurred. The child will begin to create facial highlights during this month. You may likewise begin to feel development as your infant flips and turns in the uterus. During this trimester, numerous individuals discover the sex of the infant. This is regularly done during a life systems filter (a ultrasound that checks your infant's actual turn of events) around 20 weeks.

Month (a month 13 through 16)

Your infant's pulse may now be discernible through an instrument called a doppler. The fingers and toes are very much characterized. Eyelids, eyebrows, eyelashes, nails and hair are framed. Teeth and bones become denser. Your child can even suck their thumb, yawn, stretch and make faces.

The sensory system is beginning to work. The regenerative organs and genitalia are presently completely evolved, and your PCP can see on ultrasound on the off chance that you are having a kid or a young lady. Before the finish of the fourth month, your child is around 6 inches in length and weighs around 4 ounces.

Month 5 (weeks 17 through 20)

At this stage, you may start to feel your child moving around. Your child is creating muscles and practicing them. This first development is called stimulating and can feel like a shudder. Hair starts to develop on infant's head. Your child's shoulders, back and sanctuaries are secured by a delicate fine hair called lanugo. This hair secures your child and is typically shed toward the finish of the infant's first seven day stretch of life.

The infant's skin is secured with a whitish covering called vernix caseosa. This "messy" substance is thought to shield your child's skin from the long introduction to the amniotic liquid. This covering is shed not long before birth. Before the finish of the fifth month, your child is around 10 inches in length and weighs from 1/2 to 1 pound.

Month (a month and a half 21 through 24)

On the off chance that you could peer inside the uterus at your infant at this moment, you would see that your infant's skin is rosy in shading, wrinkled, and veins are noticeable through the infant's clear skin. Infant's finger and toe prints are obvious. In this stage, the eyelids start to part and the eyes open.

Infant reacts to sounds by moving or expanding the beat. You may see jolting movements if infant hiccups. Whenever conceived rashly, your infant may get by after the 23rd week with escalated care. Before the finish of the 6th month, your child is around 12 inches in length and weighs around 2 pounds.

Month 7 (weeks 25 through 28)

Your infant will proceed to develop and create stores of muscle versus fat. Now, the infant's hearing is completely evolved. The child changes position every now and again and reacts to improvements, including sound, agony, and light. The amniotic liquid starts to decrease.

Whenever conceived rashly, your infant would probably make due after the seventh month. Toward the finish of the seventh month, your child is around 14 inches in length and weighs from 2 to 4 pounds.

This is the last piece of your pregnancy. You might be enticed to begin the commencement till your due date and expectation that it would come early, however every seven day stretch of this last phase of advancement enables your infant to plan for labor. All through the third trimester, your child will put on weight rapidly, adding muscle to fat ratio that will help after birth.

Keep in mind, despite the fact that mainstream society just notices nine months of pregnancy, you may really be pregnant for a very long time. The average, full-term pregnancy is 40 weeks, which can bring you into the 10th month. It's likewise conceivable that you can go past your due date by up to 14 days (41 or 42 weeks). Your medical services supplier will screen you intently as you approach your due date. On the off chance that you pass your due date, and don't go into unconstrained work, your supplier may prompt you. This implies that drugs will be utilized to cause you to start giving birth and have a child. Try to converse with your medical services supplier during this trimester about your introduction to the world arrangement.

Month (two months 29 through 32)

Your child will proceed to develop and create stores of muscle to fat ratio. You may see that your infant is kicking more. Infant's cerebrum is growing quickly right now, and your child can see and hear. Most inner frameworks are all around growing, however, the lungs may at present be youthful.

Your infant is around 18 inches in length and weighs as much as 5 pounds.

Month 9 (weeks 33 through 36)

During this stage, your infant will proceed to develop and develop. The lungs are near being completely evolved now. Your child's reflexes are composed so the person can flicker, close the eyes, turn the head, handle solidly, and react to sounds, light, and contact. Your child is around 17 to 19 inches in length and weighs from 5 ½ pounds to 6 ½ pounds.

Month 10 (Weeks 37 through 40)

In this last month, you could start giving birth whenever. You may see that your child moves less because of restricted space. Now, your child's position may have changed to plan for birth. In a perfect world, the infant is head down in your uterus. You may feel truly awkward in this last time span as the infant drops down into your pelvis and plans for birth.

Your infant is prepared to meet the world now.

Your infant is around 18 to 20 inches in length and weighs around 7 pounds

CHAPTER SIX

It's (at last) finished, you've been compensated with an absolutely real marvel - and another title: Mother. Grappling with your new job, while figuring out how to think about your child, can be overpowering for any lady.

Like pretty much everything else in your life, your body faces critical changes in the many months following your child's introduction to the world. In this baby blues period, which starts following conveyance, your body will recuperate from labor c, revamp its quality and start to recapture its pre-pregnancy shape.

The more you think about what's in store, the more ready you'll be to adapt to the physical and passionate changes that come post-pregnancy.

Symptoms

Ladies may encounter a wide scope of baby blues issues, some more genuine than others and each with its own manifestations. A portion of the more normal issues include:

- Postpartum contaminations, (counting uterine, bladder, or kidney diseases)

- Excessive seeping after conveyance

- Pain in the perineal region (between the vagina and the rectum)

- Vaginal release

- Bosom issues, for example, swollen bosoms, contamination and obstructed channels

- Stretch imprints

- Hemorrhoids and blockage

- Urinary or fecal (stool) incontinence

- Balding

- Post pregnancy anxiety

- Discomfort during sex

- Difficulty recovering your pre-pregnancy shape

Causes and Treatment

Baby blues Drain

Albeit some draining is ordinary following conveyance, substantial draining or discharge happens in only 2% of births, frequently after long works, various births or when the uterus has gotten contaminated.

Baby blues discharge is the third most regular reason for maternal demise in labor. It as a rule happens in light of the fact that the uterus neglects to appropriately contract after the placenta has been conveyed, or due to tears in the uterus, cervix or vagina. Not long after the child and placenta have been conveyed, you will be checked to ensure the uterus is contracting as it should. In the case of draining is serious, your maternity specialist or specialist may rub your uterus to enable it to agreement, or you might be given an engineered hormone called oxytocin to help animate withdrawals. The person in question will probably play out a pelvic test to discover the reason for the discharge, and your blood might be tried for disease and weakness. On the off chance that the blood misfortune is unnecessary, a blood bonding might be suggested.

In the event that drain starts possibly 14 days after conveyance, it might be brought about by a bit of the placenta that has stayed in the uterus. Assuming this is the case, the tissue will be taken out precisely. When you are home, report any weighty seeping to your primary care physician right away.

Nonetheless, on the off chance that you have a bump that doesn't react rapidly to home treatment, consult your PCP.

Uterine Contaminations

Ordinarily, the placenta isolates from the uterine divider during conveyance and is removed from the vagina inside 20 minutes in the wake of conceiving an offspring. In the event that bits of the placenta stay in the uterus (called held placenta), it can prompt disease.

A disease of the amniotic sac (the sack of water encompassing the infant) during work may prompt a baby blues contamination of the uterus. Influenza like side effects joined by a high fever; fast pulse; strangely high white platelet tally; swollen, delicate uterus; and noxious release for the most part show uterine contamination. At the point when the tissues encompassing the uterus likewise are tainted, torment and fever can be serious. Uterine contaminations as a rule can be treated with a course of intravenous anti-microbials, which are utilized to forestall possibly perilous intricacies, for example, harmful shock.

Infection of C-section Incision

Adhere to your medical services supplier's directions about thinking about your C-area cut. Consult your primary care physician in the event that you see indications of disease, for example, red, swollen skin or depleting discharge. Fight the temptation to scratch. Attempt cream to ease tingling.

Kidney Diseases

A kidney disease, which can happen if microorganisms spread from the bladder, incorporates manifestations, for example, urinary recurrence, a compelling impulse to pee, high fever, a by and large debilitated inclination, torment in the lower back or side, blockage, and excruciating pee. When kidney disease is analyzed, a course of anti-microbials - either intravenous or oral - as a rule, is recommended. Patients are told to drink a lot of liquids and are approached to give pee tests toward the start and end of treatment to screen for any leftover microscopic organisms.

Make certain to report any unexplained fever that creates in the early weeks after conveyance to your

PCP. This could be an indication of baby blues disease.

Perineal Torment

For ladies who conveyed vaginally, torment in the perineum (the territory between the rectum and vagina) is very normal. These delicate tissues may have extended or torn during conveyance, making them feel swollen, wounded, and sore. This uneasiness may likewise be exasperated by an episiotomy, an entry point here, and there made in the perineum during conveyance to shield the vagina from tearing.

As your body mends in the weeks following labor, the uneasiness ought to decrease. Sitz showers, cold packs or warm water applied to the zone with a spurt container or wipe can help maintain a strategic distance from disease and diminish delicacy. It's additionally critical to wipe yourself from front to back after defecation to abstain from contaminating the perineum with germs from the rectum.

In the case sitting is awkward, you might need to buy a donut formed cushion at your neighborhood drugstore to help facilitate the tension on your perineum. A remedy or over-the-counter torment reliever (non-ibuprofen, in case you're bosom taking care of) likewise can help.

At the point when you feel like it, pelvic floor works out (regularly called Kegel works out) can help reestablish solidarity to your vaginal muscles and help the recuperating cycle along. In the event that you have expanding or steady agony in the vaginal region, in any case, suspend the activity and alarm your PCP.

Vaginal Release (Lochia)

A wicked, at first hefty, release from the vagina is basic for the initial a little while after delivery. This release, which comprises of blood and the remaining parts of the placenta, is called lochia. For the initial hardly any days after labor, the release is brilliant red and may incorporate clusters of blood. The stream will in the long run help, as will its tone - progressively turning pink, at that point white or yellow prior to halting out and out. The splendid red release may return on occasion, for example, after bosom taking care of or too-incredible exercise, yet its volume by and large eases back extensively in around 10 to 14 days.

Swollen (Engorged) Bosoms

At the point when your milk comes in (around two to four days after conveyance), your bosoms may turn out to be huge, hard and sore. This engorgement will ease once you build up a bosom taking care of example or, in case you're not bosom taking care of, when your body quits creating milk (normally under three days if your child isn't nursing).

You can facilitate the inconvenience of engorgement by wearing a well-fitting help bra and applying ice packs to your bosoms. On the off chance that you are bosom taking care of, you can alleviate a portion of the weight by communicating - either physically or with a bosom siphon - limited quantities of milk. In the event that you are not nursing your infant, dodge hot showers, and communicating any milk. This will just befuddle your body into delivering more milk to redress. Oral torment relievers can assist you with persevering through the inconvenience until your milk flexibly evaporates.

Mastitis

Mastitis, or bosom contamination, typically is demonstrated by a delicate, blushed region on the bosom (the whole bosom may likewise be included). Bosom contaminations - which can be welcomed on by microscopic organisms and brought down guards coming about because of stress, weariness, or broke areolas - might be joined by fever, chills, fatigue, cerebral pain, or potentially queasiness and heaving. Any of these manifestations ought to be accounted for to your PCP, who may suggest treatment with anti-infection agents.

In the event that you have bosom contamination, you may keep on nursing from the two bosoms. Mastitis doesn't influence your bosom milk. It's additionally critical to rest and drinks a lot of liquids. Warm, wet towels applied to the influenced territory may help mitigate uneasiness; and cold packs applied subsequent to nursing can help diminish blockage in your bosom. You may likewise need to abstain from contracting bras and garments.

Stopped up Channels

Stopped up milk channels, which can cause redness, torment, expanding, or a protuberance in the bosom can mirror mastitis. Be that as it may, not at all like bosom diseases, solidified, obstructed, or stopped pipes are not joined by influenza-like side effects.

Bosom rub; regular nursing until the bosom is purged; and warm, soggy packs applied to the sensitive territory a few times each day may take care of the issue. Nonetheless, on the off chance that you have a protuerance that doesn't react rapidly to home treatment, counsult your PCP.

Stretch Imprints

Stretch imprints are the striations that show up on numerous ladies' bosoms, thighs, hips, and midsection during pregnancy. These ruddy imprints, which are brought about by hormonal changes and extending skin, may turn out to be more observable after conveyance. Despite the fact that they may never vanish totally, they will blur impressively over the long haul. While numerous ladies buy unique creams, salves, and oils to help forestall and eradicate stretch imprints, there is little proof that they work. About portion of ladies create stretch imprints during pregnancy, whether or not or not they have utilized any skin balms.

Hemorrhoids and Clogging

Hemorrhoids and clogging, which can be disturbed by the weight of the amplified uterus and baby on the lower mid-region veins, are both very normal in pregnant and baby blues ladies. Over-the-counter treatments and splashes, joined by an eating routine wealthy in fiber and liquids, typically can help decrease the stoppage and the expansion of hemorrhoids. Warm Sitz showers followed by a virus pack likewise can offer some alleviation. An inflatable, doughnut formed cushion, which can be bought at any drugstore, can help ease distress brought about by sitting.

Try not to utilize purgatives, suppositories, or purifications without asking your primary care physician, particularly on the off chance that you've had an episiotomy or have joined in the perineal region.

Urinary and Fecal Incontinence

Urinary incontinence and, less regularly, fecal incontinence, plague some new moms soon after conceiving an offspring.

The accidental section of pee, particularly when snickering, hacking, or stressing, as a rule, is brought about by the extending of the base of the bladder during pregnancy and conveyance. Generally, time is all that is required to restore your muscle tone to typical. You may rush the cycle by doing Kegel works out.

Meanwhile, wear defensive underpants or sterile napkins. On the off chance that the difficult perseveres, converse with your primary care physician, who might have the option to endorse prescription to soothe the issue. On the off chance that you experience torment or consuming or have awkward desperation to pee, tell your primary care physician. This could be an indication of bladder disease.

The absence of gut control regularly is ascribed to the extending and debilitating of pelvic muscles, tearing of the perineum, and nerve injury to the sphincter muscles around the butt during conveyance. It is generally regular in ladies who have had delayed work followed by vaginal birth.

Albeit fecal incontinence, as a rule, vanishes following a while, talk with your PCP about activities to assist you with recovering control of your insides. Fecal incontinence that doesn't resolve itself over the long run may require a careful fix.

Going bald

That radiant sheen that pregnancy brought to your hair may blur when your child is a half year old. You'll probably see balding also. During pregnancy, soaring hormones forestall the ordinary, practically indistinct day by day loss of hair. A while after conveyance (or when breastfeeding eases back or stops), numerous ladies start to fear the most noticeably terrible as they watch their hair drop out at a disturbing rate. Have confidence, the hair you're losing is just equal to the hair you would have shed during pregnancy had your hormones not stepped in. By and large, the unexpected change in hair volume is brief and not perceptible to other people.

Post-birth anxiety

Most ladies experience an instance of "postnatal anxiety" after the introduction of their youngster. Changes in hormone levels joined with the new duty of thinking about an infant, cause numerous new moms to feel on edge, overpowered, or furious. For most, this crankiness and mellow gloom disappear inside a few days or weeks.

Longer enduring or more serious misery is delegated post birth anxiety (PPD), a condition that influences 10% to 20% of ladies who have quite recently conceived an offspring. PPD, which normally becomes obvious fourteen days to a quarter of a year after conveyance, is portrayed by serious sentiments of tension or misery. Absence of rest, shifts in hormone levels, and actual agony after labor would all be able to add to PPD, making it hard for certain ladies to adapt to their new job and defeat their feeling of forlornness, dread or even blame.

The initial phase in treating post pregnancy anxiety is enrolling the help of family and dear companions. Offer your emotions with them, and get their assistance in thinking about your baby. Make certain to examine any PPD side effects with your primary care physician, who can endorse prescription or prescribe uphold gatherings to assist you with bettering adapt to these new and new feelings.

In the event that your downturn is joined with the absence of interest in the infant, self-destructive or vicious considerations, visualizations, or unusual conduct, get quick clinical consideration. These manifestations could show a more genuine condition called baby blues psychosis.

Inconvenience During Sex

You can continue sexual action once you feel great - both genuinely and inwardly. After a vaginal birth, it's ideal to delay intercourse until the vaginal tissue recuperates totally, generally four to about a month and a half (less in the event that you didn't have an episiotomy). After a cesarean birth, your PCP will most likely encourage you to stand by about a month and a half.

You may discover sex to be truly awkward, even difficult, for as long as a quarter of a year after conveyance, especially in the event that you are bosom taking care of. Since bosom taking care of diminishes levels of the hormone estrogen in the body, your vagina might be surprisingly dry during the baby blues period. A water-based ointment can help calm a portion of the distresses. Delicacy at the area of an episiotomy likewise isn't unprecedented for quite a long time or months subsequent to conceiving an offspring.

Even after your body recuperates, you may find that you are less inspired by sex than you were before your infant shown up. Actual weariness joined by new interruptions and passionate changes can negatively affect your moxie. Numerous ladies fight sentiments of ugliness in the baby blues period and some think that its more hard to accomplish climax. Bosom taking care of can likewise change how you and your accomplice see sexual closeness. Offering your sentiments to your accomplice and perceiving that these issues normally are impermanent may assist you with managing them all the more without any problem.

Recovering your pre-pregnancy shape

Exercise is perhaps the most ideal approaches to lose post-pregnancy weight recover your energy level, assuage pressure, and reestablish your muscle quality. Except if you've had a cesarean conveyance, troublesome birth, or pregnancy inconveniences (in which case, you should converse with your PCP), you can typically continue moderate exercise once you feel like it. On the off chance that you practiced previously and during pregnancy, you have a head start on baby blues wellness, however don't anticipate hopping promptly once more into an overwhelming system work out.

Energetic strolling and swimming are incredible activities and great approaches to develop to more extraordinary exercises. In view of the danger of microscopic organisms entering the recuperating tissue of the vagina, notwithstanding, you ought not swim for the initial three weeks after conveyance.

Conditioning and fortifying activities, for example, sit-ups or leg lifts, are probably the most ideal approaches to kick off your baby blues program.

Light, dull weight-lifting likewise can enable your body to get once more into pre-pregnancy shape. In any case, recollect, go slowly and center more around long haul wellbeing than on transient outcomes.

Numerous wellbeing and wellness clubs, clinics, and neighborhood junior colleges additionally offer baby blues practice classes. Notwithstanding giving extraordinarily planned activities, these classes can be an incredible method to connect with other new moms and get the help you have to stay with an activity program.

CONCLUSION

Keep on monitoring any strange changes in your body in the days and weeks after conveyance. Call your Primary Care Physician promptly in the event that you experience any of the accompanying indications. They could demonstrate a genuine baby blues confusion.

•	Vaginal draining heavier than your ordinary period.

•	Increasing or tenacious agony in the vaginal or perineal region.

•	Fever over 100.4 degrees F.

•	Sore bosoms that are hot to the touch.

•	Pain, expanding, or delicacy in your legs.

•	Hack or chest torment.

•	Pain or consuming while peeing, or a persevering and unexpected inclination to pee.

•	Nausea as well as regurgitating.

•	You feel discouraged, have an absence of interest in your child, or have self-destructive or fierce musings or mental trips.